Repurpose Your Placenta

7 Amazing Gifts From Your Baby's Afterbirth

Ruth Goldberg, CNM

Foreword by
Willow Buckley, CCH, CD (DONA) and co-author of
How to Conceive Naturally and *Have a Healthy
Pregnancy After 30*

Copyright © Ruth Goldberg

ISBN: (paperback) 978-1-772277-014-8

Cover photo of Dragon's Blood Tree by Stefan Geens with permission. www.stefangeens.com

The Dragon's Blood Tree (Dracaena cinnabari) or the Socotra tree is native to the Socotra archipelago in the Indian Ocean. It is so named for the red sap that the trees produce.

Contents

Acknowledgements   vii

Foreword   ix

Introduction: Meet Your Amazing Placenta   xiii

Chapter 1: Cutting the Cord   1

Chapter 2: Burning the Cord   9

Chapter 3: Delayed Cord Clamping   17

Chapter 4: Not Cutting the Cord (Lotus Birth)   25

Chapter 5: Cord Blood Collection   37

Chapter 6: Keepsakes and Mementos   45

Chapter 7: Ritual and Burial   53

Chapter 8: Placentophagy   63

Chapter 9: The Care and Feeding of Your Placenta   77

Chapter 10: Is That Legal?   83

About the Author   89

To anyone who has had a placenta,
made a placenta
or will have or make a placenta

Acknowledgements

Writing a book was a bucket list item for me, but shortly after beginning this project, I realized it would also be life changing.

I want to thank Raymond Aaron for his excellent 10-10-10 Program which made writing this book so simple, yet thorough.

Of course, I want to thank my husband, Steven R Blount, for his steady support. He is my Hero and I love how he worships the water I walk on. And my three children, Martin Smith, Autumn Smith and Lance Smith who have gifted me with motherhood and grandmotherhood.

I want to thank the many friends and colleagues who provided priceless feedback and assistance on the manuscript:

Annie Calderwood, a dear childhood friend

Dr Beverly Tew, Dr Kathryn Fick and Joyce Garcia, CNM all of whom I am privileged to work with

Shivam Rachana, author and passionate Lotus Birth authority. Your feedback was invaluable.

Stephan Geens, whose marvelous photo graces the cover.

Kristen Iwai, who made my professional photo shoot an absolute delight.

I have received amazing support and inspiration from:

Stephanie Dawn, Birth Goddess, professional coach and advocate,

Care Messer, childbirth educator, doula, mother and all-around extraordinary woman who sparked my interest in placentas,

Amanda Johnson, who taught me about encapsulation.

Writing this book has been an amazing experience. I can't wait to do it again!

Foreword

What is the third stage of labor? Did you know it was the release and birth of the placenta? I didn't until I became a labor doula.

In fact, most people do not consider the placenta an important part of birth, which is understood with the main event being the baby, but it is in fact the final stage of birth. Furthermore, the placenta has an incredible role during pregnancy as it nourishes the growing baby inside.

As a labor doula and homeopathic practitioner I make sure to discuss what a mother plans to do with her placenta after birth, and her postpartum plan. In regards to the placenta I often go over placenta encapsulation and keepsakes, but it usually ends there. After reading this book I have so much more to offer my clients!

As an experienced midwife, Ruth Goldberg, has taken it upon herself to create this incredible book to guide you through everything you ever wanted to know about the placenta. *Repurpose Your Placenta* is comprehensive, thorough and an example of the marriage of science and the intuition. Going beyond just the function of the placenta, Ruth takes you through the cultural, ritualistic and medicinal qualities is possesses. This book is the first of its kind.

I know that while you are planning for your baby's birth you probably did not consider how you want to use the placenta. It is not usually included in baby shower registries, or "What To Have At Home" checklists – and that is a tragedy.

My children and I have personally experienced the benefits of a few of the options in this book; delayed cord clamping, cord keepsakes and placenta encapsulation, which I must say contributed to two glorious postpartum experiences. I have also been witness to the profound importance of the placenta to other women and children around the world.

You deserve to benefit from this priceless organ too. Let's not forget that you grew it from scratch!

Read this book and include your placenta in your birth plan. Read the resources listed in this book's website www.repurpose yourplacenta.com and educate yourself about how the placenta can continue to support you and your baby long after the birth.

I believe in placentas, and, after learning how to repurpose your placenta, you will too.

Willow Buckley, CCH, CD(DONA) and co-author of *How To Conceive Naturally* and *Have a Healthy Pregnancy After 30*

Introduction
Meet Your Amazing Placenta

Birth is a seminal event in your life. You are born, you give birth, you witness birth and you may even be a birth professional. The power of birth touches us all. With each birth a transformation occurs. Everything else becomes trivial as the miracle of new life takes center stage. Pain, fatigue, tears and worries - all of these are forgotten as you, your family and your birth team revel in the arrival of the new, precious bundle.

And yet after the baby's first cries there quietly follows a seldom-celebrated arrival. The placenta- the afterbirth- is usually reviled and often discarded; however, the placenta plays a critical role in pregnancy and birth. The arrival of the placenta is usually eclipsed by the birth of your baby, but no birth is complete until the placenta has emerged as well.

From the beginning, your placenta diligently multi-tasks, protecting and nourishing both you and your baby during your pregnancy and through the birth. As you will see in the coming chapters, your placenta can continue to provide amazing gifts to both you and your baby long AFTER the birth.

During pregnancy, your baby's blood flows takes a different route through the heart and body than it does once your baby is outside the womb. Your baby's heart circulates blood throughout his or her body, largely bypassing the lungs and kidneys. While your baby's lungs and kidneys are functional in the womb, they remain relatively dormant in utero. (AHA American Heart Association, 2014) (Association of Women's Health, Obstetric and Neonatal Nurses (AWHONN), 2009)

The blood chemistry of the fetus is designed to allow the fetus to grow and thrive on much less oxygen in utero than what is needed after birth. (Association of Women's Health, Obstetric and Neonatal Nurses (AWHONN), 2009)

With the miracle of the first breath, your baby's circulation changes course through the heart and lungs and the infant's kidneys are activated. As the lungs are inflated with air for the first time, your baby's' blood chemistry changes to support life outside the womb. (Association of Women's Health, Obstetric and Neonatal Nurses (AWHONN), 2009)

Did you know that the umbilical cord (if allowed to remain intact) continues to pulse, delivering oxygen- rich blood to your baby for several minutes AFTER birth? In fact, the placenta contains approximately 100 ml -up to 50%- of your baby's total blood supply. (American Academy of Pediatrics (AAP), 2012)

Once the infant has transitioned to life outside the womb, his or her blood stops coursing through the umbilical cord and the cord itself becomes flaccid. Subsequently, as the uterus recognizes that the birth is accomplished, she contracts and the placenta peels away from the uterine wall. There is a small gush of blood as the placenta is expelled from the uterus, and the muscular walls of the uterus contract firmly, helping to staunch further bleeding. This event signals the beginning of the postpartum recovery period.

Tragically, in the US healthcare system, the placenta is usually discarded as biohazardous waste. The idea of utilizing the placenta after birth is relatively new to the United States. The purpose of this book is to present you with your options so you may include your placenta in your birthplan.

What would you do if you knew that your placenta could continue to nourish both you and your baby long after the birth? Do you know your placenta options? Do you know how to take advantage of the many gifts your placenta can provide?

The following chapters will discuss the placenta options available to ALL mothers helping you to determine which options are best for you and your baby while showing you how to take advantage of those options.

You may consider dividing you placenta into portions to enjoy more than one type of benefit, but since the placenta is a finite object, dividing it will reduce the volume of any placenta keepsake or benefit. For example, you may desire to bury the placenta (Chapter 7) but also want the umbilical cord shaped into a keepsake (Chapter 6). Or you may desire a Lotus Birth experience (Chapter 4), but also desire the benefits of encapsulation discussed in Chapter 8.

Each chapter explores a specific placenta option in depth. At the end of each chapter, the references used to compile the information have been listed. These lists can also be found at the reference page of the website www.repurpose yourplacenta.com.

PLACENTA OPTIONS

Did you know that you have options regarding what happens to your placenta after childbirth?

In most hospitals, when a woman is admitted to give birth, she is asked to sign a consent to have the placenta and other tissues disposed of by the hospital. This is a standard procedure that allows the hospital to properly dispose of "biohazardous or medical waste" such as blood samples, diseased gall bladders, etc. The placenta is included within this category of waste materials. Since these tissues or biohazardous waste products are tissues from your own body and therefore belong to you, the hospital needs your permission to dispose of them. Moreover, it is of the utmost importance for public safety that these tissues be properly disposed of in order to protect the public from disease and to keep the environment safe. If you choose to discard your placenta, your signature allows the facility to dispose of it for you.

Nonetheless, you may also request to take your placenta home and dispose of it yourself, rather than have the hospital dispose of it. If you choose one of the other options discussed in this book, it is often necessary to make your request in writing.

You may take your placenta home whether you have had a vaginal or a cesarean birth. Check with your hospital and doctor or midwife first, BEFORE you reach the last months of your pregnancy. Some hospitals require a court order to allow you to leave with your placenta, while others simply have you sign a form in advance. Some health practitioners are unfamiliar with placental options and may need more information to be able to assist you with your desired choice. Many midwives and doulas exercise these options as a matter of course. In any event, it is important to be prepared before your birth.

Each of these options can be used in any birth setting — home, hospital or birth center- and at any type of birth- whether vaginal or cesarean. For information on how to incorporate these options into a cesarean birth, please read, A Family Centered Cesarean: Taking Back Control of My Son's Birth found on this book's website, www.repurposeyourplacenta.com.

Chances are, your provider and/or the hospital or birth center has employed at least one of these options and will support you in achieving your desired choice.

In the event you encounter obstacles to keeping our placenta, Chapter 10 - "Is That Legal?" covers ways to work with your birth team to help you exercise your placenta choice.

A brief description for your placenta options and the benefits are listed here:

Option	Benefits
Discard	Your placenta provided you with your baby! There is no messy clean up nor any concern for proper transportation or storage of "medical waste"
Delayed cord clamping	Provides additional iron and blood cells to your baby. (This is especially important in premature births)
Cord blood collection	Stem cells
Lotus Birth	The benefits of delayed clamping plus a period of complete mindfulness.
Cord buming	The benefits of delayed clamping plus a ritual severance. Protects your baby from infection and bleeding from the stump
Keepsakes (drying the cord into shapes or dreamcatchers)	Provides a memento for you, your family and your baby to enjoy
Placentaphagy (Consuming the placenta) There are two options here: raw (immediately after birth) and encapsulation (preparation occurs usually within 24 hrs of birth for later use) Burial	Prevents fatigue and post partum depression. Promotes healing and pain relief. Support breastfeeding. May allow for hormonal balance during premenstrual and perimenopausal phases. Provides another opportunity for sacred ritual plus unparalleled as fertilizer
Freeze and save for later	Allows you time to decide which option is best for you or to save for later use

In the Western world, the placenta has little to no cultural value and is usually incinerated as medical waste. As healthcare providers are beginning to see an ever-increasing number of culturally diverse clientele, the need for cultural competency with regard to healthcare is essential.

For some interesting reading, you may check this book's website, www.repurposeyourplacenta.com to learn some fascinating ways other cultures view the placenta as an important part of the birth.

In the next chapter, we explore the eons-old discussion about when to cut the umbilical cord.

CHAPTER 1 – CUTTING THE CORD

The first option, discarding your placenta, was discussed in the introduction. This chapter now explores the option for delayed clamping of the umbilical cord.

Nature is amazing in her ingenuity. While in the womb, your baby has much less oxygen available than outside the womb, yet thrives nonetheless. Fetal circulation is vastly different than mature circulation. While in the uterus, the fetal heart pumps blood through structures that cause the blood to almost completely bypass the lungs and kidneys. (AHA American Heart Association, 2014) (Association of Women's Health, Obstetric and Neonatal Nurses (AWHONN), 2009)

Two structures in the fetal heart -the foramen ovale and the ductus arteriosus- allow the fetal blood to bypass the lungs.

The heart receives blood from the body through the veins and then sends it out to the body through arteries. The heart is divided into four chambers. Each chamber receives blood while the heart is in a relaxed state, then propels the blood forward to another chamber or vessel as the heart contracts. The foramen ovale is an opening between two chambers of the heart which allows the fetal blood to mix in those chambers and keeps most of the fetal blood from leaving the heart and entering the lungs. (Association of Women's Health, Obstetric and Neonatal Nurses (AWHONN), 2009)

Another structure, the ductus arteriosus is a tiny vessel that connects the aorta (the major artery that takes blood from the heart to the body) to the pulmonary artery (the vessel which transports blood from the heart to the lungs to exchange carbon dioxide [CO_2] for oxygen). Your baby makes breathing movements while in utero, an action that promotes full growth and development of the lungs. During gestation, his or her lungs are filled with amnionic fluid and are non-functioning, meaning that the lungs do not provide the CO_2/oxygen exchange for your baby. Instead, this process is accomplished through your placenta. (Association of Women's Health, Obstetric and Neonatal Nurses (AWHONN), 2009)

Another mechanism that allows your baby to thrive with less oxygen is s/he has a large amount of additional red blood cells to carry what oxygen is available. Much of this additional blood is contained within the placenta, also a reservoir for fetal blood. In fact, your placenta is estimated to contain about 100ml of fetal blood by the due date. (American Academy of Pediatrics

(AAP), 2013) (Association of Women's Health, Obstetric and Neonatal Nurses (AWHONN), 2009).

The fetal kidneys start producing very dilute urine at three months gestation. In fact, much of the amniotic fluid is provided by the fetal urine. Fetal urine is mostly water and does not contain the same waste products as mature urine. Many of the waste products that would normally be expelled through urinating are removed from your baby through your placenta. (Lim, 2010).

With the first breath, the infant's physiology shifts from fetal circulation to mature circulation. The blood flow reverses its course through the heart and is pumped into the lungs to exchange carbon dioxide (CO_2) for oxygen for the first time. The infant's blood begins flowing through the filter of the kidneys and waste is excreted as normal urine. (Association of Women's Health, Obstetric and Neonatal Nurses (AWHONN), 2009)

Remember the extra red blood cells your baby has while in growing in utero? Even if the umbilical cord is cut early, your baby's body will still have more red blood cells than s/he needs immediately at birth. Those extra red blood cells break down and are metabolized in the days following birth. A byproduct of this metabolism is called bilirubin. The accumulation of bilirubin in the baby's blood stream causes the characteristic newborn jaundice often seen in babies within the first week of their birth. This jaundice is usually harmless, but can cause brain damage if bilirubin levels become extremely high. Bilirubin is excreted through your baby's' bowel movements. Treatment for high bilirubin includes providing frequent feedings, as well as phototherapy in the form of indirect sunlight or if necessary, "bilirubin lights" provided in the hospital.

The experience of birth is as much work for your baby as it is for you. Your baby experiences the birth through the mother's body chemistry. The infant's own body is contorted and compressed through the mother's pelvis and birth canal. Ultimately, the infant is literally thrust into a different world than previously known. Suddenly, there is cold air and bright lights. Sounds are no longer muffled by tissues and fluid but clear. Sensitive skin is touched –directly- by other human beings for the first time.

This physiologic shift from life inside the womb to life outside the womb, can take several minutes to complete. The umbilical cord pulses throughout the entire pregnancy and birth, providing oxygen and nutrients to the infant from the earliest stages of gestation and for several minutes after the infant's first breaths.

Could it be beneficial to your baby to have the added support of the cord blood during this monumental shift? If an infant is premature or challenged in other ways, could the mother's body –via the umbilical cord- still support your baby for a time outside the womb? Could this be a precious, underutilized resource?

First, let's look at how the umbilical cord works in the womb. Have you ever wondered why a baby can be born with his or her cord around the neck or even knotted and still be well?

Many well-meaning friends and relatives will warn you about cord safety. They'll say, "Make sure the cord isn't around the neck" or they will claim certain activities may cause the cord to wrap around your baby's neck. This is not true.

Thirty percent of perfectly healthy infants will be born with the cord around the neck (nuchal cord) or even with true knots in the cord. How does this happen and how is your baby protected from asphyxiation?

While in the womb, your baby does not "breathe" oxygen the way we do. As previously discussed, during pregnancy most of your baby's blood actually bypasses the lungs. The oxygen is provided entirely through the umbilical cord directly to your baby's circulation. The cord looped around the neck is not strangling him - it is more like a necklace than a noose. As long as there is sufficient slack in the cord, your baby can remain well oxygenated. Your baby makes occasional breathing movements in the womb and "breathes" the amniotic fluid which plays an important role in expanding the lungs and preparing your baby for living outside the womb.

Your baby's own activities may cause the cord to knot or loop around the neck. True knots occur early in pregnancy. In the first months of pregnancy when your baby is very small and the cord is long, your baby can swim in a circle and then swim through the loop the cord makes as it follows him or her. This causes a knot to form in the umbilical cord. The infant can also wrap or unwrap the cord around his or her neck at any point in the pregnancy simply by moving and turning in the womb.

Your baby is generally well- protected from "cord accidents" in the womb. The umbilical cord has three vessels, two of which are arteries, so it has a pulse. It is turgid with your baby's blood making it more like a pulsing snake than a limp garden hose. Also, the outside of the cord is very slick -and has NO traction- so any knots tend to remain loose and the cord glides across itself and other surfaces easily. The amniotic fluid is mostly water, but with a slippery consistency that lubricates your baby and cord and provides a significant amount of cushioning for your baby and cord. These layers of protection provide a safe environment for your baby to move while keeping the cord safe from compression, even if the cord becomes entwined with your baby.

In the Western world it is common to clamp and cut the umbilical cord immediately after birth. Some claim that this practice came about due to time constraints placed on medical staff in busy hospitals, or because early cord clamping could reduce the amount of linens that were soiled at a birth. More realistically, however, this practice became common due to the belief that early cord clamping would reduce hemorrhage in the mother and jaundice in the infant.

According to Goer and Romano, authors of Optimal Care in Childbirth: The Case for a Physiologic Approach, the strongly held belief is that labor and birth are dangerous for both mother and baby. As a result, the notion that immediate intervention is necessary gives rise to the practice of early cord clamping as an act of rescue. This belief- that early cord clamping is necessary to promote breathing in the infant, to prevent an overload of red blood cells in the infant, to facilitate newborn resuscitation, to release the cord around your baby's neck as s/he is born or to permit a sample of blood to be drawn from the cord- is not supported by science. Yet these practices persist today.

The contemporary practice of cord blood banking also supports the rationale for early cord clamping. Cord blood banking is covered in Chapter 5.

There is NO research or evidence to suggest that routine early cord clamping is necessary or beneficial to either your baby or you. An alternative method is to delay cutting the cord until it has stopped pulsing. This is known as delayed cord clamping and there is strong clinical evidence that this method benefits your baby with no risk to you. (American Academy of Pediatrics (AAP), 2013). Before we discuss delayed cord clamping in Chapter 3, let's take a look at another way to severe the umbilical cord – burning the cord.

CHAPTER 2 – BURNING THE CORD

Severing the cord is a significant event in the birth experience. Not only when but how to sever the cord is an important decision. There are three options for severing the cord: clamp and cut, cord burning and not severing the cord, a practice called "Lotus Birth." Lotus Birth is explored in Chapter 4.

CLAMPING AND CUTTING

Clamping and cutting is the most recognizable form of severance. Once your baby is born, the cord is clamped in two places. Then the cord is cut between the two occlusions with scissors, a knife or other cutting device. The purpose of clamping twice is to prevent blood loss from your baby through the cord vessels and to prevent hemorrhage in the mother. The concern for maternal hemorrhage does not bear out in the evidence.

The remaining cord stump usually dries and hardens- like a scab- and falls off the baby's abdomen in 3-5 days, leaving an adorable scar we know as the belly button. This approach has many benefits such as ease and safety, but what if you desire another way to acknowledge your baby's entry into the world? What if there is another way?

Some have adopted the practice of cord burning.

UMBILICAL CORD BURNING

Now, take a breath, this is not as dangerous and out there as it sounds. The history is sketchy, but it seems cord burning was instituted in disaster areas and areas where resources are scarce as a means to prevent cord infections. Cord infections are very rare in the US because we have easy access to sterile instruments and medications. But in disaster areas, (such as Thailand after the 2004 tsunami), burning the cord became an important means to protect babies from cord infections.

Cord burning has since become an important ritual to acknowledge your baby's transition from the womb to world. The ritual poses no risk your baby and - according to some- provides additional health benefits to your baby.

According to holistic health teachings, the umbilicus provides an entry place to all abdominal organs. Burning the cord drives the vital life force (qi) into your baby and provides invigorating health benefits.

According to Dr. Joseph Kassel, ND, LAc. (who also serves on the Volunteer Medical Advisory Board for Mother Health International), burning the cord allows the following:

"The flame brings the yang qi from the placenta and fire energy into the baby. It has an ethereal and remarkable effect on the baby. It is the core. The umbilicus is the entry place to all abdominal organs. By heating the cord and driving the last of the blood through there you are giving a profoundly tonic treatment for the baby who has just run a marathon…. Cord burning reduces the risk of bleeding and entry of infections. You are warming digestion which will reduce the tendency for jaundice, besides just creating a strong baby which means a good nurser."

Warming the digestion will reduce the tendency for jaundice and promote breastfeeding. Cord burning also believed to prevent anemia by preventing babies from reabsorbing iron and eliminating it through the bowel.

Cutting the cord can be described as sterile, medical, violent and too hasty in proportion to the magnitude of the birth event. Cord burning requires a little time and preparation and mental focus, during which you, your family and other participants can celebrate, give thanks, or otherwise reflect upon the birth of your baby. It is a more mindful, even sacred way to acknowledge your baby's arrival earthside.

Many home birth midwives and alternative birth centers routinely include cord burning in the birth plan. These are the most welcoming places to burn the umbilical cord. Hospitals usually do not allow open flames or even burning incense due to local fire safety regulations.

Materials:
Two taper candles or a long stem lighter/s
Barrier for baby (cardboard/paper plate wrapped in tin foil)
Small fire/heat tolerant bowl or burning box

Basic Instructions:
- Allow the placenta to emerge with the cord intact after the birth of your baby
- Swaddle the infant with the cord exposed
- While your baby sleeps or breastfeeds, hold the barrier against his abdomen and exposing the cord
- Place the limp cord through the notches in the burning box or drape the cord over a bowl
- Hold the lighted candles or the lighter UNDER the cord and inside the bowl until the cord is cauterized and severed
- Allow the cauterized end of your baby's cord to cool before allowing it to touch your baby

The remaining stump will be longer than usual (about 6 inches or so) but this is not a concern for your baby's health or wellbeing.

The burning process can take up to 15 minutes to complete which allows time for a self-made ceremony if you desire.

Other suggestions are:

- Sing, chant, pray/give thanks or remain silent/meditate
- Talk to your baby and describe what is happening, present him/her with their name, allow siblings to welcome your baby
- Read to your baby

Basic Outline for a Sacred Cord Burning Ceremony

1. Prepare the space. Turn off ALL cell phones and electronic equipment. Close/lock doors and leave a "Do Not Disturb" sign outside. Select the lighting, music, incense you desire, if any. Include any sacred items to keep you focused and in the moment. (figurines, icons, sigils, photos, artwork, books, other mementoes) Gather the cord burning item listed above. Position yourself and your baby comfortably and safely with the umbilical cord exposed.

2. Prepare for the burning of the cord. Once you and your baby are comfortable and safely positioned (safety first, last and ALWAYS!) set the flame protection in place along with the firesafe container for the burning to take place. Keep the remaining cord and attached placenta in another firesafe container

3. Invoke the Deity of your choice. Then light the candles.

4. Give your offerings. As you watch the cord burn, direct your love and attention to your baby and offer your best wishes for your baby's health and fulfillment.

5. Protect the cauterized ends of the cord. At the moment the cord separates, place your baby's end in the burning container until it is cooled, or hold it above any surfaces to allow it to cool. Place the placenta end in the firesafe container with the placenta.

6. Give thanks. Give thanks to the Divine and all those who brought this baby and birth to you.

7. Close the ceremony and properly dispose of all used materials.

Some parents choose not to cut the cord at all. They keep the baby, cord and placenta intact in the days following the birth. This practice called "Lotus Birth" is explored in the following chapter. Read on to learn how to achieve this safely (and neatly).

CHAPTER 3 – DELAYED CORD CLAMPING

The debate about when to cut the umbilical cord has been raging for centuries.

Aristotle, a Greek philosopher known as "The Father of Modern Science," studied animals (because dissecting human cadavers was punishable by death) and described his findings in Historia Animalium. In this work, Aristotle describes how the cord should be tied once the placenta had "come away" from the mother and how the midwife could strengthen a weak baby (or even resuscitate a baby) by -"milking"- the cord blood towards the baby.

Erasmus Darwin grandfather to Charles Darwin, was an observant scientist and physician. In his published work, Zoonomia, he strongly advocates for delayed cord clamping:

Another thing very injurious to the child is the tying and cutting of the navel string too soon, which should always be left till the child has not only repeatedly breathed but till all pulsation in the cord ceases. As otherwise the child is much weaker than it ought to be, a part of the blood being left in the placenta which ought to have been in the child and at the same time the placenta does not so naturally collapse, and withdraw itself from the sides of the uterus, and is not therefore removed with so much safety and certainty.

John Whitridge Williams, the recognized leader of academic obstetrics in the United States published his first textbook, Obstetrics in 1903. In its earliest editions, he wrote:

The question as to the proper time for tying the cord has given rise to a great deal of discussion. Formerly it was the custom to ligate immediately after the birth of the child; but Boudin 1875 showed that 92 cubic centimeters more blood escaped from the maternal end of the cord after early than after late ligation, thus indicating that that amount was lost to the fetus by early, and saved for it by late ligation...

Williams continues:

I have always practiced late ligation of the cord and have seen no injurious effects following it, and therefore recommend its employment unless some emergency arises which calls for earlier interference.

Williams penned six editions of his textbook during his lifetime. Subsequent editions continue to acknowledge the controversy of early versus delayed cord clamping and support delayed cord clamping to some degree.

Proponents of delayed cord clamping cite that allowing the cord to pulse 30-60 seconds (or even longer) can provide the infant with many benefits. This time allows for your baby's physiology to stabilize and to help determine when to sever the cord.

When delayed cord clamping is employed, your baby rests skin-to-skin with you on your abdomen or- if the cord is long enough- at your breast. Your body temperature can therefore warm your baby. You and your baby may then be covered with a receiving blanket to further retain heat. Your baby's vital signs can easily be monitored throughout this progress.

Another method called, "milking" the cord, was studied in preterm infants and found to be equally effective in providing the placental transfusion of blood to the preterm infant. The authors concluded that milking the cord of the preterm infant four times was equal to delaying cord clamping for 30 seconds. This could be a valuable option in circumstances in which severing the cord sooner is desirable. (Rabe & al, February 2011)

A pediatrician, Dr Alan Greene passionately promotes delayed cord clamping. In his video-TICCTOCC (Transitioning

Immediate Cord Clamping To Optimal Cord Clamping)- a TEDx Talk in Brussels in 2012, Dr Greene recommends delaying cord clamping for 60-90 seconds to allow the optimal autotransfusion of the infant's blood from the placenta and cord into the infant. This video can be found in the Free Downloads page of www.repurposeyourplacenta.com and on Dr Greene's website www.drgreene.com.

Others recommend waiting until the cord stops pulsing altogether. This could take up to five minutes or more.

All mammals, in fact, are born with a pulsing umbilical cord. In nature, mothers wait for the pulsation to cease before severing the cord. In circumstances where both you and your baby are well and you are willing and able to hold your baby, delayed cord clamping is safe and uncomplicated.

Delayed cord clamping allows for more of your baby's red blood cells to enter his or her body, thus reducing the incidence of anemia. More white blood cells are transfused as well which helps to strengthens your baby's immune system and protect him or her against infection. In addition, more stem cells are saved for the infant's use to build and repair tissues. The skin-to-skin time promotes bonding and breastfeeding plus it allows you, your partner and baby time to integrate the birth experience. (Greene, 2012)

Premature infants face many challenges. These include anemia, infection and intracranial hemorrhage –bleeding inside the brain.

The World Health Organization (WHO) recognizes that delayed cord clamping may provide newborns with additional protection from anemia for up to six months after birth. The WHO endorses delayed cord clamping, especially for infants born in "low-resource areas with less access to iron-rich foods."

In December 2012, the American Congress of Obstetricians and Gynecologists (ACOG), published a Committee Opinion acknowledging that delayed cord clamping in preterm infants has clinically demonstrated benefits of reducing intracranial hemorrhage by 50 percent. That same month, that same document was endorsed by the American Academy of Pediatrics (AAP). The AAP also publishes and promotes specific resuscitation protocols for newborns which birth professionals are required to learn.

Delayed cord clamping is not currently part of these protocols. In fact, the procedures for resuscitation of ALL infants suggest that the cord be cut almost immediately upon birth in order to move the infant to where the resuscitation equipment is located.

Angie Evans, a Canadian doula and prenatal educator, writes in an article published in Midwifery Today (2012) that neonatal resuscitation guidelines in many countries –Canada, Australia, Europe and the United Kingdom- incorporate delayed cord clamping in their neonatal resuscitation procedures. Angie notes that the American guidelines do not suggest a time period for severing the cord at all. She also writes of an innovative infant resuscitation device called BASICS (Bedside Assessment Stabilisation and Initial Cardiorespiratory Support) which is designed to conduct infant resuscitation with the umbilical cord intact. One of the inventors, Dr Andrew Weeks, states that "it is crazy that the most vulnerable babies are born and whisked off and surrounded by a scrum of doctors."

At the time of this writing, studies are underway at Liverpool Women's Hospital to determine the efficacy of this device and the resuscitation of vulnerable infants with the umbilical cord intact.
(http://public.ukcrn.org.uk/search/StudyDetail.aspx?StudyID=14 007)

Sharp Mary Birch Hospital for Women in San Diego is leading the way with this technology. See this news video for more information
http://fox5sandiego.com/2014/11/18/new-technology-at-sharp-mary-birch/.

Another fascinating method of newborn resuscitation is placenta stimulation or heating the placenta. (Lim, 2010)

Among the traditional midwives of India and Bangladesh. Some resources report that the lotus style of birth is common among the traditional midwives. (The Jeeva Project, 2014) (The Matrika Project, 2014) When a baby is born limp and lifeless or stressed, the midwives will wait for the placenta to emerge and place it into a bowl of warm water or massage it. The traditional midwives report that this often revives the baby. (Lim, 2010) (The Jeeva Project, 2014) (The Matrika Project, 2014)

Using the placenta to resuscitate the baby has not been well studied. In light of the evidence that keeping the cord intact can benefit your baby, there is hope that keeping the cord intact at the time of birth could become a common part of newborn care.

The above discussion begs the following question - if the placenta is still functioning and providing support to your baby in the immediate time after birth, then one must ask "why cut the cord at all?" That concept is discussed in the next chapter on Lotus Birth.

CHAPTER 4 – NOT CUTTING THE CORD

Your baby is born. The cord is cut. Your precious infant is weighed, measured, medicated, bathed, diapered and swaddled then returned to you. For many in the Western world, this is the standard protocol at birth. Boxes checked. Papers signed. Job well done. Mom and baby home in 24 hours.

But what if there is another way?

According to some, this clean and efficient protocol after birth actually interferes with the bonding process and induces a severance greater than that just between infant and the placenta.

The phrase, "Peace on Earth begins with birth," comes to mind here. How we do birth, is how we do everything. How we tend to mothers and babies at the moment of emergence is how we treat the vulnerable, the helpless. It's how we nurture ourselves and others. The way we conduct birth demonstrates how we conduct our lives. The way we are present at birth is the way we value what is precious and sacred to ourselves and to others.

Lotus Birth (also known as umbilical integrity or umbilical non-severance) is the practice of keeping the infant, cord and placenta intact until the cord dries and separates itself, usually 3 to 10 days after birth. Is a means to ensure your baby receives the full benefits of delayed cord clamping and causes you-the parents- to be fully mindful of how you handle your baby in those first days. It demands the parents slow down for a period of days fully and mindfully integrate the birth experience. This time is often referred to as a "baby moon".

In the paradigm of Lotus Birth, the cord and placenta – as living tissue – is considered an appendage of the baby. To severe the cord, before the baby is ready to release it, is to commit an act of violence, an amputation. Part of the Lotus Birth ritual is to allow the baby to release his placenta in his own time.

Lotus Birth has no science behind it. No randomized controlled studies exist. It is not an evidence-based practice. In fact, the only authority to comment on the practice is the Royal College of Obstetrics and Gynaecology whose position statement advises parents to be on the lookout for infection in the infant because the placenta contains blood (organic material) and can become a source of infection.

So, where did this idea come from and why would anyone want to do it?

On the heels of the Women's Liberation movement and sexual revolution of the 1970's came a greater awareness about birth. Prior to this time, it was common practice to anesthetize a woman at the point of birth and remove her baby with forceps after cutting a large episiotomy (an incision made to widen the vaginal opening). The newborn was held upside down and spanked into taking his first breath. The woman was then introduced to her baby about 24 hours later.

Fathers were not allowed into the delivery room and were only allowed to see their babies through a glass window in the nursery. Breast-feeding was strongly discouraged both culturally and by the medical profession.

During the 1950's to 1960's a few physicians, namely Lamaze, Grantly Dick-Read and Laboyer begin to question the birth practices of the time and designed alternatives which centered around the experience of the woman, the father and the baby.

The women of the 1960's no longer accepted the traditional, passive role while in childbirth. They practiced psychoprophylaxis, the practice of using breathing techniques and a focal point to achieve an unmedicated birth. Women who used these methods spoke of the deep satisfaction and empowerment they felt regarding the birth experience. Their babies were born alert and vigorous. Their babies did not need resuscitation from drugs administered to their mothers nor a slap on the bottom to begin breathing. "Natural birth" and "birth without violence" became the buzzwords in the birthing community.

Women of the 1970's began to take greater ownership of their bodies. These women began to explore and question health practices of the time. They became fiercely resistant to any external, paternalistic influences on their bodies, their sexuality, reproduction or the birth experience. Women reclaimed their autonomy.

Woman centered birth classes, freestanding birth centers, homebirth and waterbirth emerged as therapeutic and safe alternatives to the hospital birth.

The search for ever greater empowerment and spiritual satisfaction in the birth experience continued.

Enter Lotus Birth.

Claire Lotus Day was a nurse and clairvoyant who claimed she could see the "auras" or energetic fields which surround all of us. She made an association between the "astral vibration of the umbilical cord being severed" and the vibration she observed when one was in a negative state. Claire began to question the need for cutting the umbilical cord. Her search for alternatives led her to Jane Goodall's work with primates. She learned that chimpanzees would give birth and keep the placenta and cord intact until it fell off on its own some days later. She chose to become pregnant in order to have that birth experience and was able to find the support to achieve that. She also researched and wrote about how to care for the baby and placenta until the "breaking forth" of the cord, her term for the time when the dried umbilical cord released from the baby's navel.

The ritual was then discovered and promoted by late midwife, herbalists, author, birth activists and mother of six Jeannine Parvati Baker. Janine chose a Lotus Birth for her last three children.

She writes," I chose to follow this ritual birth process because of the primary understanding of the incredibly vital link which exists between mother and baby. Lotus Birth is a demonstration that all attachments, to placenta, to mother, to earth, will eventually cease of their own accord."

Jannine describes how practicing Lotus Birth causes the family and their friends to slow down and honor and integrate the birth experience and the new life that has joined the earth.

Your baby is kept in skin-to-skin contact with the mother at all times. Moving with your baby-placenta unit requires a degree of effort and awareness. Visits from friends and family are kept to a minimum. Only the most open-minded are welcome or willing to visit while the placenta is still present.

Another proponent of Lotus Birth, Dr. Sarah Buckley is an Australian physician, author and birth activist. She wrote about how she was drawn to the idea of Lotus Birth after meeting Shivam Rachana, author of Lotus Birth: Leaving The Umbilical Cord Intact. Dr. Buckley describes the Lotus Birth experience of each her last three children on her website. She writes:

Lotus birth has been, for us, exquisite ritual that has enhanced the magic of the early postnatal days. I notice and integrity and self-possession with my lotus-born children, and I believe that lovingness, cohesion, to Mother Nature, and trust and respect for the natural order of all been imprinted on our family by our honoring of the placenta, the Tree of Life.

A PDF of Dr Sarah Buckley's Lotus Birth protocol can be downloaded from this book's website www.repurpose yourplacenta.com.

Robin Lim, an American woman and midwife who was CNN's Hero of the Year for 2011, operates the Bumi Sehat birth center in Indonesia. Known locally as Ibu or "Mother" Robin she provides free medical care to mothers and babies of the region who otherwise would not be able to afford care.

In her book *Placenta: The Forgotten Chakra*, Ibu Robin describes how she is able to attend 10 to 20 Lotus Births annually. She describes how to care for your baby's little companion comfortably and safely:

- Once the placenta is born, place it into a bowl and clean it with clear water to thoroughly wash away blood and clots
- Pat it dry and place the placenta spongy side up (This is the red meaty side that was attached to mothers uterine wall)
- Salt it generously, making sure the salt is in all the folds
- Wrap the placenta in cloth and place it spongy side down in a basket. A basket is better than a bowl because it allows air to circulate. This helps prevent a rotting odor in addition to the salting
- Then generously salt the shiny side of the placenta (this is a site where the cord attaches)
- Place the whole package next to your baby. Always be mindful of pulling or tugging your baby's cord
- Change the placenta cloth every few hours as it will absorb moisture from the placenta

Ibu Robin also describes adding herbs to the salt mixture such as rosemary or lavender.

The salt and herb mixture can be re-applied daily to promote the drying of the placenta and cord. The cord dries and stiffens on its own and will release from the umbilicus 3 to 6 days.

Ibu Robin also describes how Lotus Birth is easily accomplished with cesarean births. The cooperation and understanding of the surgeon and hospital staff is essential. Perhaps gently stating your desires and preparing the hospital staff well in advance is a means to achieving a Lotus Birth with vaginal or cesarean births in the Western world.

Leaving the cord and placenta attached to your baby for days after the birth is certainly not a common birth ritual in the Western world. Indeed, the mere mention of the ritual will bring up fears about infection, biohazardous waste and the mental stability of the parents.

Let's look at these issues.

Infection

Neonatal Tetanus - According to the World Health Organization (WHO) fact sheet on the subject, neonatal tetanus is a form of generalized tetanus in newborn infants who do not have protective passive immunity because the mother is not immune. *It usually occurs through infection of the on-field umbilical stump, particularly when the stock is cut with unsterile instruments.* (Italics mine). Neonatal tetanus is estimated to kill over 200,000 newborns each year. These deaths almost always occur in developing countries. Neonatal tetnus is very rare in developed nations.

The fact sheet continues to state that neonatal tetanus can be prevented by providing for sterile instruments and maternal vaccinations, neither of which are readily available in disaster areas or other areas with limited resources.

Perhaps another means to prevent infection is to burn the cord or to separate a few hours after the birth when the drying and closure of the umbilical vessels is completed.

Lotus Birth could protect babies from neonatal tetanus because the cord is not severed.

Biohazardous waste

Although the placenta is very much alive the time of the birth, it begins to die shortly after the infant has transitioned to life outside the womb. Because the placenta contains blood and is comprised of organic material, it is an ideal breeding ground for microbes. This deserves consideration.

By liberally salting the placenta, frequently changing the cloth that wicks away fluid and allowing air to circulate around the placenta, microbes are deprived the moisture needed to thrive. Growing microbial colonies are also responsible for the foul odors associated with rot and disease. The salting and drying of the placenta creates a hostile environment for microbes thus minimizing unpleasant odors. The herbs also create a pleasing scent, but cannot mask rot.

When the placenta is released, it can be buried under a tree or rosebush. Returning the placenta to the earth is an important means to complete the placenta's lifecycle. Burying the placenta is explored in Chapter 7.

Parents also have the option to sever the cord shortly after the birth and then encapsulate the placenta. Placental encapsulation as discussed in Chapter 8.

Mental stability

The parents who choose Lotus Birth are not making an uninformed choice. Nor are they careless of the placenta and baby. In fact the reality is quite the opposite.

The mother of Lotus Birth, Claire Lotus Day educated herself of the possibilities and designed a safe method to manage the placenta. She chose to birth this way because of the benefits she believed her baby would derive from maintaining the entire fetal-placenta circuit. There are no long-term studies or in-depth research currently available regarding Lotus Birth. Therefore, one must rely upon anecdotal evidence.

I questioned my midwife friends, doulas and other birth workers who have had clients who chose Lotus Birth. My question was "Have any of your Lotus Birth clients experienced any negative effects, such as infection, bleeding or even just having a disappointing experience?"

The answer was a unanimous "No."

That said, the absence of serious conditions occurring with lotus born babies DOES NOT equal safety.

In the same mental health vein, there is a curious phenomenon called "placenta trauma". Placenta trauma is the painful physical and emotional experience of having one's placenta violently severed and removed. Babies are observed to cry, startle and clinch their fists when the cord is clamped and cut. The results of this severance range from a sense of incompleteness to rebirthing memories of a violent amputation.

A prominent psychohistorian, Lloyd deMause, is featured in Shivam Rachana's is book, *Lotus Birth: Leaving the Umbilical Cord Intact*. DeMause associates the root causes of historical events, such as war in childbearing practices. DeMause theorizes if the woman is toxic and the entry into the world is violent, we produce children who will become toxic, violent adults who play out their traumas in an attempt to resolve them. He associates the toxic womb and violent birth experience with the way countries wage war.

The work of Lloyd deMause and the other authors noted above are also featured in the publications of The Association of Prenatal and Perinatal Psychology and Health (APPAH) and organization dedicated to the education of professionals and the public about the lifelong impact of pregnancy and birth on individuals, families and society. A link to APPAH and the work of deMause can be located on this book's website, www.repurposeyourplacenta.com.

No matter how you choose to handle your baby's placenta, many families find that saving the baby's blood - which is contained in the cord and placenta -a valuable resource. You can read more about this innovative option in the following chapter.

CHAPTER 5 - CORD BLOOD COLLECTION

On the coattails of stem cell research has come the practice of cord blood banking. Many families and individuals have benefited from the use of banked cord blood and many more are encouraged to have their baby's cord blood banked in case the baby or another compatible family member has a need for it.

Is cord blood banking for you? How does it work and is it truly useful?

All our tissues are composed of microscopic cells. These cells are specialized for the tissue they comprise; liver cells make the liver and its functions, brain cells make the brain and its functions, etc. Most cells are specialized and not interchangeable, therefore, when cells of any organ are damaged, they must be regenerated by that organ or we must learn to function without them. Some organs like the brain and spinal cord CANNOT regenerate damaged tissues. This is where stem cell research becomes important.

Stem cells are cells which have not yet differentiated, so they have the potential to become any type of tissue. They are generic cells, anatomic play-doh that can morph into many types of cells. The umbilical cord is a rich source of stem cells and parents may choose to bank their newborn's cord blood and/or umbilical cord itself against the possibility that it will be useful in the future, should the child or a compatible family member have a disease that is treatable by cord blood stem cells.

It is important here to note that the placenta contains two types of stem cells: hematopoietic stem cells (HSC) and mesenchymal stem cells (MSC). Hematopoietic stem cells are found in fetal blood and adult bone marrow. These stem cells have tremendous potential to treat numerous diseases of the blood such as leukemia, lymphoma and some anemias. Research also suggests that genetic disorders of the immune system and certain metabolic abnormalities could be treated as well.

Mesenchymal stem cells are found in large numbers in the substance which surrounds the umbilical cord vessels, known as Wharton's jelly and amniotic fluid. Mesenchymal stem cells, in theory, have the capacity to differentiate into many other types of cells; neuron, muscle and cardiac, pancreatic and liver cells for example.

While transfusions of hematopoietic stem cells have been used successfully worldwide, the potential for using mesenchymal stem cells is controversial. According to recent (2013) lectures given at the International Cord Blood Symposium, the potential exists to create many tissues from MSCs, however, that potential has yet to be realized.

While any adult can consent to donating his bodily tissues, harvesting fetal cells is an important ethical issue.

Stem cells are present in great quantities in fetal blood. One the baby is born, the fetal blood is still pulsing in the cord can be collected before the cord is severed- much like a blood donation - and the harvested cells can be used for research, donation for a specific patient, or frozen and saved for future use. Collecting fetal blood through the umbilical cord is not painful for the baby because there are no nerve endings in the umbilical cord. It is also safe to collect fetal blood from the umbilical cord after it is clamped because babies are usually born with more blood than they will need once they are outside the womb.

The most common method requires the cord be clamped and cut first. Once the umbilical cord is cut, a needle is inserted into the umbilical vein usually while the severed cord is still pulsing and the placenta is still attached to the mother. The remaining fetal blood is collected into a bag which is attached to that needle.

Cord blood collection is most successful if it is done while the cord is still pulsing. This means that waiting for the cord to stop pulsing after the birth could reduce the amount of fetal blood cells collected.

The collected cord blood is then "cryopreserved" or frozen for later use.

There are two options for where to store your baby's cord blood: public cord blood banks and private cord blood banks. Public cord blood banks store cord blood and tissues for the benefit of the general public. They are supported by the medical community.

Private cord blood banks store your baby's cord blood for the exclusive use of the baby or family members. These private companies charge hefty fees for their services ($2000 - $3000 to start, then $100+ annually).

In the United States, the Food and Drug Administration regulates how human cells and tissues are collected and stored by public and private companies. New York, New Jersey and California also require additional accreditation.

Public and private cord blood banks can voluntarily register with the American Association of Blood Banks (www.aabb.org) or the Foundation for the Accreditation of Cellular Therapy (www.factwebsite.org).

Canada has the Canadian Blood Services (www.blood.ca) and in the United Kingdom, the Human Tissue Authority (www.hta.gov.uk) regulates cord blood banking.

The American Academy of Pediatrics (AAP) 2007 Policy Statement on Cord Blood Banking states that:

"Physicians should be aware of the unsubstantiated claims of private cord blood banks made to future parents that promise to insure infants or family members against serious illnesses in the future by use of the stem cells contained in cord blood."

After the first sibling-donor cord blood transplant was performed in 1988, the National Institute of Health (NIH) awarded a grant to Dr. Pablo Rubinstein to develop the world's first cord blood program at the New York Blood Center (NYBC) in order to establish the inventory of non embryonal stem cell units necessary to provide unrelated, matched grafts for patients.

For parents, private storage at birth of stem cells from both cord blood and cord tissue offer more options for future medical use.

Currently there is no standard procedure or accrediting criteria for storage of MSC from umbilical cord tissue. Many cord blood banks are storing the cord tissue by freezing an intact segment of the umbilical cord. This procedure has the advantage of waiting for the technology of cell separation to mature, but has the disadvantage that there is no guarantee it will be possible to efficiently retrieve viable stem cells from a previously frozen cord. A few cord blood banks are extracting stem cells from the cord tissue before cryogenic storage. This procedure has the disadvantage that it uses the current separation method, but the advantage that it yields minimally manipulated cells that are treatment ready and comply with FDA regulations on cell therapy products.

The Controversy

An in-depth discussion of the ethical and medical/legal aspects of cord blood and stem cell therapies is beyond the scope of this book. What follows is a brief description of a few of the controversies surrounding cord blood banking.

- While there is much general support in the medical community for public cord blood banking, the option of private banking has raised questions. According to a paper published in the journal *Biology of Blood and Marrow Transplantation* in March of 2008, lifetime probability (up to age 70) that an individual in the US would undergo a stem cell transplant using your own stem cells (autologous) is 1 in 435, the likelihood of an allogeneic transplant from a matched donor (such as a sibling) is 1 in 400, and the overall likelihood of any type of stem cell transplant is 1 in 217.

- Many types of tissue transplants are dependent upon the recipient making a genetic match with a donor. According to the National Marrow Donor Program the likelihood of finding a donor is greater if you are Caucasian. Patients of mixed ethnic origin are more challenged finding a match. This suggests that families of mixed ethnic origins could strongly benefit from cord blood banking.

- Using autologous stem cells to treat genetic disorders is counterproductive, since the stem cells will contain the same genes which caused the disorder. This suggests that the stem cells saved from an infant who later develops leukemia, for example, would not be suitable for transplant to himself or another.

Parents make many important decisions before the birth of their child. Cord blood banking is a very personal and unique choice many parents may find comforting.

If cord blood banking is not for you, then you may consider preserving a part of the placenta as a keepsake. Read on to Chapter 6 – Placenta Keepsakes to explore how this can be done.

CHAPTER 6 - PLACENTA KEEPSAKES

The precious moments in our lives are many, but fleeting. Since we cannot hold memories in our hand, or keep them in a jar, we find substitutes. Tangible items that we imbue with the meaning of the moment. No one leaves Disneyland without at least one souvenir. We press dried flowers into books, safe concert tickets, collect spoons or symbols from around the world, we even preserve the ashes of loved ones. Entire industries are devoted to preserving our memories: scrapbooking and Shutterfly for example.

The birth of our children is undoubtedly one of those many precious moments. We take countless pictures and email them to friends and relatives and post on social media. We also save little mementoes from the birth; the name bracelet from the hospital, the first receiving blanket and we even preserve the gown that they wore when they were baptized.

Believe it or not your placenta can be one of those keepsakes. Here are your options for handling the placenta:

DISCARD

This is the traditional way to handle a placenta in the Western world. If you find handling the placenta distasteful, you may choose this option.

When a placenta is discarded in the hospital it usually is sent to pathology in a bag or small container. It is held in a refrigerator until such time it is incinerated along with all the other medical waste. There will be no ceremony, no marker and no notification.

Midwives who attend births at home or in a free-standing birth center also release the placentas to a medical waste company should their clients choose not keep them.

There is no shame in discarding the placenta. It has met its purpose and you may have no further need for it. Unless you choose to use the placenta after your birth, discarding it is a safe and healthy way to handle the placenta.

FREEZE

If you are undecided or wish to utilize your placenta at a later date, you may take your placenta home and freeze it. Double bag your placenta in large plastic storage bags or place it into a freezer safe container. You can keep you placenta frozen for up to six months if you plan to consume it or indefinitely if you plan to bury it.

It is important to note that the longer the placenta is frozen the more of its vitality is lost. Mothers who plan to consume their placenta in any way are strongly encouraged to have it prepared as soon as possible after the birth. Check with your placenta professional to see how long she recommends your placenta be stored before preparation.

When you thaw your placenta, you cannot use a heat source. No ovens, or microwaves allowed! This will destroy the tissues of the placenta and render your placenta inert. Allow your placenta to thaw naturally in the refrigerator for about 24 to 48 hours.

Some guidelines of how to store your placenta after the birth are summarized here: (Placenta Professionals, 2014)

Immediately upon the birth of the placenta-	
At home	Refrigerate immediately
In a Birthing Center	Place the placenta on ice in a small lunchbox size cooler and once home place the placenta into the refrigerator
At a Hospital	Place the placenta on ice in a small lunchbox size cooler and have your designated "placenta person" immediately remove the placenta from the hospital and place it into your refrigerator

Optimal Timeline for Placenta Care and Preparation	
Birth to 4 hours	Your placenta can be prepared fresh and will produce the most benefits at this point. You can eat the placenta raw; make placenta herbal essence, placenta herbal tincture, placenta homeopathic remedy; utilize the Traditional Chinese Medicine placenta preparation and encapsulation.
4 to 48 hours	Your placenta must be refrigerated at 4 hours postpartum, and the placenta can still be prepared fresh. At this point you can eat the placenta raw; make placenta herbal essence, placenta herbal tincture, placenta homeopathic remedy; utilize the Traditional Chinese Medicine placenta preparation and encapsulation.
48 hours to 2 weeks	Your placenta must be frozen at this point. It takes 24 – 36 hrs for the placenta to thaw in the refrigerator prior to preparation. At this point you can make placenta herbal essence, placenta herbal tincture, placenta homeopathic remedy, the resulting solutions may be less effective by using a frozen placenta and will continue to lose effectiveness the longer the placenta being used has been frozen; utilize the Traditional Chinese Medicine placenta preparation and encapsulation, still retaining many of the benefits.
2 weeks to 4 weeks	Your placenta can still be encapsulated, but the longer it is frozen, the less effective it may become
1 month to 6 months	Your placenta can still be encapsulated. However, the longer the placenta is frozen the less benefit it has to the mother, and the more at risk the placenta is to freezer burn.

PLACENTA KEEPSAKES

Prints. Many placenta professionals will make prints of the placenta on acid-free paper. The placenta is placed upon a flat surface. The cord can be arranged in to an initial, a heart or a spiral shape if the parents desire. The paper is pressed firmly onto the placenta and the blood stains the paper in the form of the placenta. One the blood dries, the placenta print can be framed as is, painted or other mediums added to embellish the image.

Cord keepsakes. Other common keepsakes are shapes made from drying the cord. While the umbilical cord is still moist can be fashioned into heart shapes, spirals, initials, even dreamcatchers. The substance which surrounds the vessels inside the umbilical cord, known as Wharton's jelly, contracts when exposed to the air and hardens as the umbilical cord dries. A simple Google search will bring up countless images of these keepsakes.

The umbilical cord can be dried into a keepsake or charm for the baby to use a special occasions. According to Cornelia Enning, author of *Placenta: The Gift of Life:*

In Europe and Africa the dried cord was kept underneath the child's pillow or tied to the bed. In Tanzania the cord is tied with a long black piece of cotton string, which remains wrapped around the baby's neck for 10 days. One Amazon tribe turns the cord into a bracelet decorated with beads to be chewed on when teething. The Australian natives make necklaces from the cord for the children who wear them for protection from disease (2007).

Keepsakes can also be designed to be kept in a man's wallet or pocket or a woman's purse.

Amnion keepsakes. The dried amnionic sac can also be the source of a very unique keepsake. Enning describes how:

If the baby is lucky enough to be born in the caul (with the membranes intact), the parents will keep a small piece of the amniotic membrane. They stretch the skin to be dry and pain symbols from religion, astronomy and nature onto the parchment like tissue later. In Islamic countries parents most commonly choose "The Eye of Fatima. " Where in Christian countries a picture the child's patron saint is very popular. Delicate pieces of amnion are set in a pendant for arm and leg bracelets. (Enning, 2007)

One artist in particular, Alison Brierley (http://alisonbrierley.wordpress.com) will make a keepsake form your placenta for a commission. Her fascinating website has images of her unique creations from placentas.

Another artists, Christina Cole (Together Again) and Amanda Johnson (The BirthRoom), can use parts of the dried umbilical cord, placenta or breastmilk and place them into beautiful beadwork to be worn as jewelry. These artists can also make beautiful keepsakes with a loved ones' cremains. Links to these artists' websites can be found at www.repurpose yourplacenta.com.

If you desire a placenta keepsake, please contact a placenta specialist before the birth of you baby to make arrangements for your keepsake.

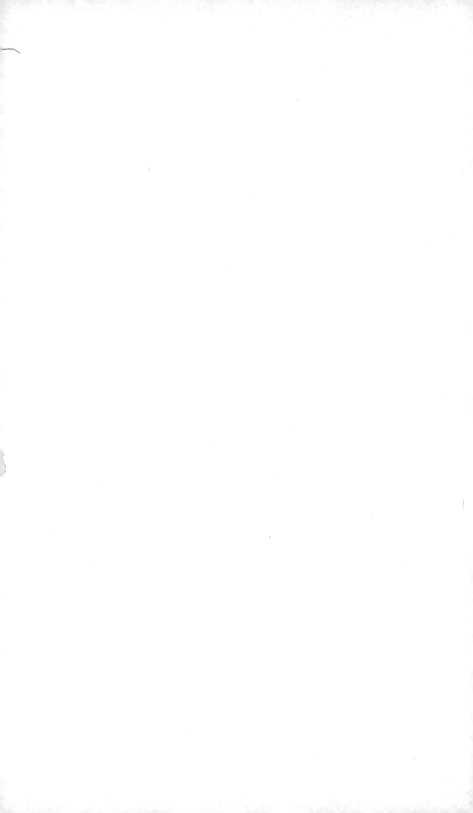

CHAPTER 7 - BURY THE PLACENTA IN CEREMONY

Many cultures place the placenta in a jar or other container and bury it to ceremoniously honor its spiritual role for the baby and family. The Maori artist Nathan Manos has created examples of this in his artwork (Spirit Wrestler Gallery, 2014).

Cornelia Enning, author of *Placenta: The Gift of Life*, identifies numerous cultural burials of the placenta. She writes,

> Our ancestors believed that a part of the child's soul stays with the placenta. Even if the placenta was born it performed its function as a root, ... -and as fertile soil. This is why it was never to be taken too far away from the child. The tree planted on top of it had to be in the immediate vicinity of the house.

> In the cities, hiding the placenta underneath one's house used to be safer. The father usually buried it immediately after the birth, either in the basement or in an adjoining building, so the household could benefit as much as possible from the placenta's fertile powers. In some areas a girl's

placenta was buried to the left of the front door, a boys to the right. It was to be kept out of reach of animals and people or the fertility of the couple and other family members was endangered. As long as the placenta stayed within the surroundings of the person it belonged to, no ill fate would befall him or her.

In 18th-century Germany and France the newborn was to be smart and well -behaved in life- if the placenta was very close to living quarters immediately after birth. Because throwing away the placenta is believed to lead to infertility in the mother, this method was sometimes used as an attempt at birth control.

In Sudan the placenta is viewed as the child's mental duplicate and is buried in a place that represents the parents' hopes and wishes for their baby. A Sudanese woman is said to have buried her son's placenta close to the medical faculty of University of Khartoum, wanting him to become a doctor!

In many cultures of the world the custom of burying the placenta is still alive today. From the people of the Andes to the Indonesian cultures, burying the placenta under the home in a specially formed pot is still common practice. Just like the German women of the 17th and 18th centuries, these women are concerned about the child's soul suffering a painful loss by being separated from its nurturing, life-giving organ. Such pain was believed to impair the child's entire future development.

Research shows research shows that many cultures believe the placenta deserves special handling due to a belief that the way the organ is handled can influence an aspect of the mother or baby's life (Young & Benyshek, 2010).

Many parents who choose to bury their baby's placenta may also freeze it until an optimal time; a certain date or occasion, or when they move to a larger house, for example. Some choose to bury it as part of a naming ceremony or the baby's first birth day or when the family moves from an apartment to a house.

Parents may purchase an eco-friendly placenta planting kit from Birth to Earth (birth2earth.myshopify.com). The kit includes a biodegradable container for the placenta, a keepsake about the event and a copper tag to place upon the tree or bush planted over the placenta to identify its unique connection to your baby.

The Birth to Earth website includes information about tree meanings and instructions on how to successfully plant a tree over a placenta.

You may choose to bury your placenta in ceremony. This is a beautiful and sacred way to acknowledge and thank the placenta for bringing you your baby and for observing your family ties to the Earth. If you choose a ceremonial burial for your placenta, see http://www.moondragon.org/parenting/placentadisposalrituals.html or http://www.marythunder.com/SpiritualServicesEvents/AnnualWomensDance/TheCordCeremony.html for suggestions.

You may choose to bury your baby's placenta at a Naming Ceremony. Of course parents are allowed to create their own ceremony to meet their own spiritual needs. However other cultures already have long-standing rituals around the naming of the baby. You may wish to borrow from these traditions while planning your baby's naming day or even utilize the rituals as they are.

The Jewish religion has a long-standing naming ceremony for baby boys and a modified one for baby girls (Cohen, 2014; Ritual Well, 2014).

Our God and God of our ancestors, sustain this child for his/her father and mother. Let her be called in Israel _____ son/daughter of _____ and _____. May the father rejoice in his offspring and may his/her mother rejoice in the fruit of her womb. Let your parents be happy; let she who bore you rejoice. Give thanks to God; God's mercy is constant. May this little one, _____, be big. As he/she has entered into the covenant, so may he/she enter into a life of Torah, loving relationships and good deeds

The Mormon Church also has an established baby naming ceremony for its families and newest members (Church of Jesus Christ of Latter-Day Saints, 2010)

Every member of the church of Christ having children is to bring them unto the elders before the church, who are to lay their hands upon them in the name of Jesus Christ, and bless them in his name" (D&C 20:70). In conformity with this revelation, only worthy men who hold the Melchizedek Priesthood may participate in naming and blessing children. *The ordinance of naming and blessing children requires authorization from the presiding authority.*

When blessing a baby, men who hold the Melchizedek Priesthood gather in a circle and hold the baby in their hands. When blessing an older child, brethren place their hands lightly on the child's head. The person who gives the blessing:

1. Addresses Heavenly Father.
2. States that the blessing is given by the authority of the Melchizedek Priesthood.
3. Gives the child a name.
4. Gives a priesthood blessing as the Spirit directs.
5. Closes in the name of Jesus Christ.

After the blessing, a church record is made for the baby and the parents receive a Blessing Certificate as a keepsake.

Because birth is a visceral, primal and ancient event linking us to eons of ancestors, some parents may prefer a more pagan ritual (Wigington, 2014).

In this ceremony, the parents take on the role of High Priest and High Priestess. It is their chance to dedicate themselves and bind themselves to their child, and swear an oath to the new baby. It is their opportunity to tell the child that they will protect her, love her, honor her, and raise her to the best of their abilities.

Hold the ritual outside, if weather permits. If that's not an option, find a place big enough for everyone you've invited. You may wish to consider renting a hall. Consecrate the entire space beforehand -- you can do this by smudging if you like. Place a sturdy table in the center to use as an altar, and put whatever magical tools you normally use upon it. Also, have on hand a cup of milk, water or wine, and blessing oil.

Invite all the guests to form a circle, filing in sunwise around the altar. If you normally call the quarters, do so now. The Guardians should take a place of honor beside the parents at the altar.

Call upon the gods of your tradition, and ask them to join you in the naming of the child. If the child is a girl, her father or another male family member should lead the ceremony; if the baby is a boy, his mother should preside.

All of the above ceremonies share the gathering of friends and family to acknowledge the blessed arrival of the baby by evoking the Divine and providing a Blessing on the infant. You may need other items as your situations requires; candles, incense, music, indoors or outdoors, etc. However you choose to design your baby's naming ceremony, you may include an acknowledgement of the placenta as the bridge that brought this life to yours.

FERTILIZER

If you choose to bury your placenta with or without ceremony, you can use it as fertilizer. It is common to bury your placenta under a rose bush or fruit tree or even in a garden plot. The placenta is organic material and contains large amounts of protein which translates into superior nourishment for the soil.

Many gardeners choose to use blood meal to nourish their garden soil. Blood meal is usually made from cow blood collected during the butchering process and then dried and crushed into power to be blended into the soil.

Assuming the placenta is similar to blood meal for soil, and the instructions for Miracle Gro blood meal can also be used for placentas, here are some recommendations for using your placenta as fertilizer:

- Dry and crush your placenta into powder
- One placenta can provide nourishment to approximately 60 square feet of soil.
- It is generally not recommended that you plant your entire placenta under one plant nor use it in a planter because the nitrogen content can be too strong for many plant roots.
- Rake or mix into the top 1-3 inches of soil
- Apply evenly around plants. Do not concentrate near the trunk or crown of the plant.
- Water after application
- You may follow with applications of blood meal every two months starting in the spring

If you choose to bury your whole placenta under a tree or other plant please check with your local nursery to determine if it is suitable for that type of plant.

Diane Bajus, midwife and herbalist located in Phoenix , Arizona recommends digging the hole an extra six inches deeper and placing the placenta at the bottom. Cover it with a layer of rocks and soil before placing the plant in the hole.

As you complete your birth plan be sure to include your placenta. For a quick guide to your placenta options see the free download "What Can Your Placenta Do for You?", also located at www.repurposeyourplacenta.com. There, you may also find a placenta specialist through the links to International Placenta and Postpartum Association (IPPA) and Placenta Benefits Inc (PBI) who can help you make the most of your placenta choices.

CHAPTER 8 - PLACENTOPHAGY

EAT the Placenta!? EWWW!! Do People Really Do That!?

Yes.

There, I said it. Many normal, healthy, SANE, educated and stable women consume their placentas. Willingly. Eagerly. By choice.

Why would anyone want to do that? It sounds gross! Isn't that cannibalism? Is that even legal?

I'm so happy you asked! Please read on! (And, yes, it is legal. Please see Chapter 10)

First, let's explore the uncomfortable ideas about this nutritional choice.

Placentophagy -or eating the placenta- is very common among most mammals. Cattle, horses, dogs, rats and non-human primates, to name a few, are all known to consume the placenta. Curiously, camels, llamas, alpacas, vicunas, guanacos and humans are among the few mammals noted to not regularly consume the placenta (Benyshek & Young, 2010). Common theories about why some mammals consume the placenta include; cleaning the nest site to prevent predators from detecting offspring, a desire for meat products after the birth, general hunger or hunger for specific nutrient found in the placenta (Benyshek & Young, 2010; Kristal, 1980; Soykova-Pachnerova, 1954).

One researcher, Mark B Kristal, PhD, of the Department of Psychology, State University of New York at Buffalo, challenges these theories and has produced evidence to point out their inconsistencies (Kristal M. B., 1980). In his research, Kristal concludes, "we have proceeded on the assumption that placentophagia has a single, fundamental, biological advantage to all mammals, such as in effect on immunology or mother infant bonding" (Kristal M. B., 1980).

Placentophagy can be considered a form of self-cannibalism, according to Kristal, DiPirro and Thompson (2012). And there are a number of psychological disorders with symptoms that include ingesting non-food items. Included in these disorders is pica, a common behavior noted in pregnancy. It is well documented that pica can represent a nutritional deficiency the pregnant woman is trying to correct. Iron deficiency is often considered the cause of pica in pregnant and non-pregnant people (MedlinePlus, 2014).

One definition of pica is the consumption of something that is not food – and in large quantities on a regular basis (Brynie, 2011). The human placenta does not meet this criteria and is not included in lists of common non-food items ingested by those with pica (Brynie, 2011; MedlinePlus, 2014).

So why in the world would a woman want to eat her placenta?

This question has not been well researched over the years, so much of the research available on this subject is many decades old. More current research has been conducted by Daniel Benyshek, a University of Nevada Las Vegas anthropologist and Sharon Young, a doctoral student of anthropology. They asked 189 women who consumed their placentas why they did it, what kind of preparation they preferred and if they would do it again (Benyshek, Cantor, Selander, & Young, 2013).

The results showed that the women perceived three positive effects: improved mood, improved energy and improved breastfeeding (Benyshek, Cantor, Selander, & Young, 2013). In general, the women reported the experience of consuming the placenta was positive and they would do it again (Benyshek, Cantor, Selander, & Young, 2013). This UNLV study is not the first to note these positive effects of consuming the placenta.

IMPROVED MOOD

Between 5% and 20% of women experience depression in the weeks after giving birth (Corwin, 2005; Yim, 2009; Yonkers, Vigod, & Ross, 2011). The high incidence of postpartum depression has prompted much research into the cause and treatment of this condition. However, no single cause of postpartum depression has been identified. Nor has any single hormone been identified as the cause of postpartum depression. Rather it is a number of factors that converge to cause postpartum depression. These factors have been identified as:

- a decline or fluctuation in reproductive hormones such as estrogen and progesterone which can predict depression in susceptible women;
- previous experience of depression and anxiety; a personal or family history of depression; marital dysfunction; and younger motherhood;
- acute stressors, including events specific to motherhood (e.g., child care stressors) and other stressful events (e.g., death of a loved one);

- exposure to toxins; crowding; air pollution; poor diet; low socioeconomic status; and low levels of social support;
- the stress of a new child, in combination with the incongruity between the expectations and reality of motherhood;
- difficult infant temperament through erosion of the mother's feeling of competence as a caregiver. (American Psycology Association, 2014; Yonkers, Vigod, & Ross, 2011; Yim, 2009)

Although hormonal changes in a woman's body associated with birth and breast-feeding could contribute to postpartum depression, no single hormone has been identified as the cause postpartum depression.

An in-depth discussion of the role of hormones in mood disorders is beyond the scope of this book. It is important to know, however that hormones do not work alone. The pituitary gland and hypothalamus in the brain, thyroid gland in the neck and adrenal glands which sit on top of the kidneys and ovaries or testicles all form an axis. Hormonal changes in any part of this axis signals the other parts to response with additional hormonal changes. The menstrual cycle is an example of how this axis functions. When all parts are functioning at their best, the woman has a regular, predictable menstrual cycle.

During pregnancy, the placenta also produces hormones to support the mother and fetus. One hormone produced by the placenta during pregnancy is called Corticotropin -Releasing Hormone (CRH). Corticotropin -Releasing Hormone is also made in the part of the brain called the hypothalamus and is an important part of the communication that occurs between the brain and adrenal glands, which sit on top of the kidneys. Corticotropin-Releasing Hormone is also considered to be an important factor in the cause of depression in the non-pregnant state. Many depressed, non-pregnant patients will show an increased sensitivity to CRH levels and may require higher CRH levels to stabilize their mood.

The CRH produced by the placenta (pCRH) is almost identical to the CRH produced in the hypothalamus (hCRH). When the hypothalamus releases hCRH, the adrenal glands are signaled to release cortisol, a hormone associated with stress. The increase in cortisol, then signals the placenta to release pCRH into the mother's bloodstream.

The placenta is known to increase the levels of pCRH in the mother in the last trimester of pregnancy. After the birth, pCRH levels decline sharply. One theory suggests that the sudden decline in the blood levels of pCRH after the birth could contribute to postpartum depression (Yim, 2009; MA Magiakou, 1996).

Women who consumed their placentas perceive that the placenta preparation they are using is stabilizing their hormone levels and thus preventing postpartum depression (Benyshek, Cantor, Selander, & Young, 2013).

Currently, women who are diagnosed with depression or other psychiatric disorders during pregnancy or after birth are treated with talk therapy and medication. It is unclear how much of an impact – if any- these medications have on the fetus or the breast-feeding infant. Physicians are advised to weigh the risks versus the benefits for each individual case. (American Congress of Obstetricians and Gynecologists, 2008). The use of placental preparations for the prevention or treatment of postpartum depression has not been empirically tested. To quote one study, "The results of such studies, if positive, will be medically relevant. If negative, speculations and recommendations will persist, as it is not possible to prove the negative" (Kristal, DiPirro, & Thompson, 2012).

IMPROVED ENERGY

Even the most well prepared and supported parents will experience exhaustion in the weeks and months following the birth of their newborn. The increase in energy needed to provide care for the newborn, disturbed sleep patterns and the physical demands of healing after giving birth can tax both parents to their limits. Anemia and fatigue in the weeks after birth are both noted to contribute to postpartum depression (Beard, 2005; Corwin, 2005).

Fatigue is a common symptom of anemia which is usually treated with iron supplementation. It is been observed that women who are not clinically anemic but experiencing fatigue will still benefit from iron supplementation (Verdon, 2003).

Women who consumed their placentas perceive they were consuming nutrients which prevent anemia and / or provide higher levels of energy during their post partum recovery (Abrahamian, 2011).

IMPROVED BREASTFEEDING

An article written in 1917 notes how consuming the placenta can ease postpartum symptoms and improve breast-feeding. The author describes how the placenta can be prepared as a meal or it can be dried and made into pills. A French midwife, Louise Toussaint, is quoted as saying "...that even in non-pregnant women and in virgins the milk secretion may be made to appear by simple placental feeding" (Unknown, 1917). In a more contemporary study, rats that consumed their placentas after delivering a litter had higher levels of prolactin, a hormone that supports lactation (Blank & Friesen, 1980). This phenomenon was also observed in a European study of human mothers who consumed their placentas (Soykova-Pachnerova, 1954).

Women who consume their placentas perceive that the placenta preparation is supporting their lactation (Benyshek, Cantor, Selander, & Young, 2013).

PAIN RELIEF

Another benefit of consuming the placenta is pain relief. Both the amniotic fluid and the placenta are known to contain a chemical called placental-opioid enhancing factor (POEF) (Kristal M. , 2008; Kristal, DiPirro, & Thompson, 2012). Studies show that the POEF raises the pain threshold in rats. Even non-pregnant rats and male rats receive this benefit from POEF (Kristal M. , 2008).

Women experience pain during post partum recovery even after the easiest of births. The breasts swell with fluid to accelerate lactation. New mothers will have muscle aches from the exertion of birth and possibly from having their legs up in stirrups for the duration of the birth. The uterus continues to contract strongly after birth in order to staunch bleeding and to return to its normal size and shape. These contractions are known as after pains and become sharper during breastfeeding sessions. Other discomforts of pregnancy such as hemorrhoids, varicose veins and pelvic pain can continue into the post partum recovery time.

Women who consumed their placentas perceive that the placenta preparation they are using can bring pain relief to ease their post partum recovery (Benyshek, Cantor, Selander, & Young, 2013).

Other benefits perceived by women who consumed their placentas are; decrease in postpartum bleeding, faster recovery, weight loss, prevented or relieved headaches, facilitated bonding with the infant, treated or prevented hypothyroidism, replenishment or regulation of hormones, increased or improved duration or quality of sleep, uterine involution, increase libido (Benyshek, Cantor, Selander, & Young, 2013)

PREPARATIONS

Some women choose to consume the placenta raw. They either consume it shortly after the birth or mix a part of it in a blender as a smoothie (Abrahamian, 2011). Since this requires immediate access to the placenta, this option is best utilized for home births.

Encapsulation is the most preferred preparation among women who consume the placenta (Benyshek, Cantor, Selander, & Young, 2013; Abrahamian, 2011). To prepare the placenta for encapsulation the placenta is first washed clean of any blood clots or debris. The cord, membranes and vessels are then carefully removed and the remaining meaty tissue of the placenta is steamed or boiled with herbs intended to enhance the placenta benefits. This is known as the Traditional Chinese Medicine method (TCM). The placenta can also be prepared as is, without steaming or herbs. The placenta is then thinly sliced and dried in a dehydrator. The dried strips of placenta are then crushed into a powder that is placed into gel capsules.

It's important to note that researchers consider the benefits of the placenta to be destroyed in the cooking process. For example it is known that POEF is inactivated by temperatures above 40°C (Kristal, DiPirro, & Thompson, 2012).

The finer points of how a placenta should be prepared, consumed and for which purpose is beyond the scope of this book. Other common preparations are tinctures, chocolates, creams and salves

Please seek a placenta specialist in your area to determine which, if any, placenta preparation is right for you. You may find a placenta specialist in your area on this book's website www.repurposeyourplacenta.com under the Placenta Services tab.

Traditional Chinese Medicine also has a use for the dried human placenta. Known as *zi he che* it is consumed as a tea and intended to revitalize the body (TCM Treatment, 2014).

Human and animal placentas have been used in cosmetic products for many years. The protein and hormonal derivatives are used as active ingredients in skin creams and hair conditioners (Cosmetic Ingredient Expert Review Panel, 2002).

The controversy over the actual medicinal benefits of the human placenta rages on. Can the experience and perception of thousands of post partum women be wrong? Will science find any evidence of therapeutic benefits of placentophagy?

Without solid, clinical research, the questions surrounding the safety and efficacy of consuming the placenta will not be answered. And who will conduct the research if there is little to no financial profit to be gained?

In the words of Arthur Schopenhauer: All truth passes through three stages: first it is ridiculed. Second it is violently opposed. Third, it is accepted as self-evident.

Websites for more information:

Independent Placenta Encapsulation Network - https://www.placentanetwork.com/

The Association of Placenta Preparation Arts - http://www.placentaassociation.com/

International Placenta & Postpartum Association – http://www.ippatraining.com/

Placenta Benefits.info - http://placentabenefits.info/

CHAPTER 9 - THE CARE AND FEEDING OF YOUR PLACENTA

What is the placenta and what does it do?

When the egg and the sperm unite inside the fallopian tube the result is called a "zygote". The zygote then floats down the Fallopian tubes into the womb. It continues to divide into four, then eight, then sixteen cells. By day three, the fertilized egg has sixteen cells and is called a morula. By day five, the morula nestles itself snugly into the rich lining of the uterus to begin growing into a fetus.

Each cell of the fertilized egg contains ALL of the new person's genetic information. Because ALL of our cells contain ALL the genetic information we need to become a human being, the cells respond to external cues which trigger the DNA to respond in specific ways, which then, in turn causes the cells to grow and differentiate into a full-fledged human baby.

When the morula lands in the lining of the uterus, the portion of the cell lining which comes into contact with the uterine wall automatically knows to start forming a placenta, which will support the pregnancy and nourish the baby. The parts of the morula which are directed away from the uterine wall form the bag of waters (amnionic sac) with the fetus inside.

The developing fetus has its own food supply which lasts for the first few weeks of pregnancy. At three weeks of pregnancy, enough placental tissue has formed to allow the baby to be nourished by the mother via the placenta.

Both the zygote's cells that contact the uterus and the layers of cells inside the mother's womb combine to form the placenta. The placenta is comprised of glandular tissue and blood vessels and is designed by the mother's physiology. The umbilical cord, which is the conduit for the blood vessels between the placenta and the baby, is designed by the baby.

Nutrient and Waste Exchange

Normal growth of the placenta depends upon the nutrients available in the uterine lining and maternal circulation. Protein fibers anchor the placenta to the uterus. In the first weeks of pregnancy the placenta literally "takes root" in the inside lining of the uterus. Tiny blood vessels grow from the placenta and corkscrew themselves into the uterine lining. Numerous small "lakes" of maternal blood form around these tiny vessels, which float like waving stalks of seaweed in these lakes. These lakes are where the nutrient/waste exchange is made between mother and baby. Amazingly, mom's and baby's blood never mix. The nutrient and waste exchanges are made via the delicate, one-celled wall of the tiny vessels. (Zhao, 2010)

Hormone and Immune Functions

The placenta also provides hormones to mom which are essential for a healthy pregnancy. In fact, your common drug store pregnancy test is designed to detect one of those hormones. (The pregnancy test is not looking for a baby, it's looking for a placenta!)

The placenta also allows the mother's immunities to pass to the fetus, starting at five months, while simultaneously protecting the fetus from the mother's immune system so s/he is not attacked as foreign DNA. What an amazing safety feature!

The umbilical cord is approximately 22-24 inches long and contains two arteries and one vein. The arteries bring blood from the baby to the placenta to expel wastes and carbon dioxide (CO_2). The vein brings nutrients and oxygen (O_2) from the mother's circulation through the placenta to the baby. The vessels of the umbilical cord are surrounded by a substance called Wharton's Jelly and wrapped in the same tissue as the bag of waters.

Our regular veins and arteries contain muscle tissue that contracts and dilates to meet physiologic demands. Placenta vessels do not contain muscle tissue; therefore, constriction and dilation are influenced entirely by hormones. (Zhao, 2010)

It's clear the placenta is a busy, multi-tasking organ. Like other organs, the placenta needs to be properly fueled in order to perform its many tasks.

We are bombarded daily with the most current research on nutrition for specific organs and tissues; calcium for bones, iron for the blood, iodine for the thyroid. What fuels and nourishes the placenta? This information is surprisingly absent in professional literature.

A strong, healthy placenta will provide hormonal support to the mother during pregnancy and nourish and protect the fetus. In the event the mother chooses to encapsulate her placenta, a vibrant placenta will provide optimal benefits.

What the placenta does determines what nourishment it needs.

Willow Buckley, a doula, certified homeopath (www.balancingyourhealth.com) and co-author of *How To Conceive Naturally* and *Have a Healthy Pregnancy After 30* with nutritionist Christa Orecchio of the Whole Journey (www.thewholejourney.com) recommends the following in a pregnant woman's diet:

- Clean protein to build strong tissue– oily fish, raw nuts, dark green leafy vegetables, miso
- Clean fat for antioxidants and cholesterol to build hormones– olive oil, fish oils, flax seed oil
- Complex carbohydrates to provide vitamins, minerals and fuel for hard working cells– fresh, organic fruits and vegetables

It should come as no surprise that the placenta needs the same nourishment as the mother and fetus!

Now that you have worked so hard to make a beautiful, healthy placenta and baby, what if you want to take the placenta home too? Can you do it legally? In front of everybody?

YES!! You Can!

Turn to the next chapter and learn about the legal aspects of keeping your placenta.

CHAPTER 10 - IS THAT LEGAL?

You and your baby made this placenta. You decide to keep it. At the birth, you are shocked and dismayed to learn that the hospital labels the placenta as "biohazardous waste" and refuses to release it to you to take home. The hospital administration claims the right to refuse on the grounds that the placenta contains blood and therefore it is unsafe to allow it to be released to the public. It must be incinerated with all the other biohazardous waste.

All you careful planning and hopes for a burial, keepsake or encapsulation are dashed.

Can they do this? Can a hospital refuse to release a placenta?

The official legal answer is "It depends." (LIFELIBERTYLAWYER, 2013)

Many states have placenta specific laws regarding how to handle the placenta. A list written, researched and maintained by Courtney Durfee (http://www.cddoula.com/) is on the book website www.repurposeyourplacenta.com.

It's a safe bet that most mothers who choose to keep their placenta are able to do so without much difficulty. The staff and providers for homebirth or a free standing birth centers are quite familiar with placenta options and might offer giving the placenta to you as part of the birth plan.

If you give birth in a hospital, you are strongly encouraged to plan ahead. You might need to meet some administrative requirements in order take home your placenta. It may be as simple as signing a release or you might need to contact a funeral director to obtain permission. (Placentas are human tissue. Some locations require this step for any human remains to be released or moved from one point to another). Many women have taken the step of obtaining a court order to release their placenta if the hospital where they choose to give birth has a strong policy against releasing placentas.

The possibilities are too numerous to explore in this book and nothing in this book is to serve as legal advice on any subject. Please consult your local placenta specialist for more information about how to keep your placenta.

Jodi Selander, doula, placenta professional and owner of Placenta Benefits.info (PBi) (www.placentabenefits.info) was instrumental in establishing a placenta friendly environment in Nevada. In 2007, one of her clients gave birth in a local hospital and was not allowed to take her placenta home. Subsequently, she and others joined forces to petition the state to allow women to keep their placentas. The story is described in the professional journal Midwifery Today (Selander, The Placenta Encapsulation Movement, 2014). If you sign up for the PBi Newsletter, you will receive access to articles and helpful tips about obtaining your placenta from a hospital.

If you desire to keep your placenta and you plan a hospital birth, it is wise to prepare well in advance so you are not disappointed at the birth. If you plan to give birth at home or a free standing birth center, be aware of the local hospital policies. In the event you need to give birth in the hospital it will serve you to be prepared.

QUALIFICATIONS OF PLACENTA PROFESSIONALS

What qualifies one to be a placenta professional? Where does one go to be educated and certified?

There are currently three organizations which provide online placenta preparation courses and certification; The Association of Placenta Preparation Arts (APPA), International Placenta & Post Partum Association (IPPA) and Placenta Benefits.info (PBi). IPPA also offers live courses worldwide.

All three organizations teach many methods of placenta preparation and require strict adherence to Occupational Safety and Health Association (OSHA) standards for safety. Placenta professionals are held to rigorous food safety and sanitation standards and a detailed code of ethics.

In general, if you decide to engage the services of a placenta professional, you will;

- You will have a personal, if not face-to-face interview to determine your needs and expectations
- You will discuss fees
- You will provide the placenta to your specialists at the time of the birth
- Your placenta preparations will usually be completed and returned within 24 to 48 hours
- Each placenta is prepared individually. Placenta professionals do not do "batches"
- The equipment used for placenta preparation is used exclusively for placenta preparation
- All equipment and surfaces are cleaned and sanitized with a bleach solution before and after each placenta is prepared

There are some circumstances which make the placenta unsuitable for encapsulation or other preparations. For example, if the placenta is not properly refrigerated and stored, if the mother is a heavy smoker or taking certain drugs. These issues will be discussed at your interview.

Please visit the websites for The Association of Placenta Preparation Arts, International Placenta & Post partum Association and Placenta Benefits.info for more information. There you will find more detailed information about their services and directories for specialists in your area.

Links to all these organizations are located at this book's website, www.repurposeyourplacenta.com and the URLs are listed in the references at the end of this chapter. If you are looking for a placenta specialist in your area or desire to become one, please go to one of these organization's websites for more information.

Thank you for choosing to read this book!

I hope you found many new and fascinating facts about your placenta options. Whether you are preparing for your own birth or you are in a birth profession, there are many facts and resources to help you appreciate the placenta. My best wishes to you and your birthing future!

About the Author

The entire birthing process has always fascinated me and, now, I have the privilege of attending women during pregnancy and at the time of birth. "Midwife" is not just my job title, it's who I am.

I have attended births both in and out of the hospital and I am eager to teach women about their magnificent bodies and how they work.

Our intuitive knowledge of birth combined with established science can produce the richest birth experience. I am dedicated to bringing the intuitive, holistic knowing of the ancients supported by evidence to provide care to women of all ages.

Ruth Goldberg is a Certified Nurse-Midwife and lives in Flagstaff, Arizona with her husband.